SUPER RICH NON PERISHABLE SURVIVAL FOODS TO STOCKPILE

Quick Guide to the Best Foods to Store for Improved Immune System and Health Care

WILFRED WILSON

copyright@2020

Table of Contents

CHAPTER ONE

INTRODUCTION

Foods can become scarce and very expensive during tough times (such as natural disasters, pandemics, wars etc). However you can choose to get yourself fully equipped by storing and preserving super rich foods at home that will improve your immune system as well as your general health care.

WHAT ARE NON-PERISHABLE FOOD

Non-perishable foods are foods that stay steady and safe to eat for extensive stretches of time without refrigeration. We as a whole realize various foods ruin at various rates.

Milk and eggs will ruin immediately left out on the counter. While a granola bar may most recent half a month with no evil impacts.

The fact of the matter is:

There are limits in food waste rates and the non-perishable things are on the furthest finish of the range. The farther, the less perishable it is.

Presently, in fact no food is genuinely non-perishable FOREVER. In the long run, all foods will get ruined, become malodorous, or lose their flavor.

Microscopic organisms will in the end deteriorate all natural issue. It takes care of off calories similarly as we do. It changes food's taste, shading smell, and can make food borne ailments whenever ingested.

Without a doubt, with the assistance of innovation non-perishable foods may most recent a very long while. Yet, don't anticipate that anything should last any longer than that.

WHY CHOOSE NON-PERISHABLE

Since you know what non-perishable foods are – you might be pondering – so what? We have refrigeration, correct?

- Non Perishable Food for Emergencies

Even though you have refrigerator, what happens when the power goes out for a couple of days or even half a month? Those solidified steaks, containers of eggs, and your head of lettuce are in a tough situation.

Furthermore, when those get ugly – you'll be happy you kept some non-perishable foods in your wash room.

Non perishable foods are a staple inside the more extensive classification of endurance food units.

Hence in this book, you will be learning spotlight on accumulating food for crises. Be that as it may, there are different motivations to put resources into non-perishable foods:

- Non Perishable Food for Camping

Some of the time it merits getting some non-perishable food for an outdoors trip. Why? Since you can abstain from managing a cooler and softening ice.

It appears as though every time I take a cooler outdoors, we purchase lunch meat and whelps. What's more, every time the ice dissolves and the ham cuts and whelps end swimming. Making a gross crude meet cesspool.

Rather, you can stay away from this whole disaster by taking a perishable meat decision like Beef Jerky.

- Non Perishable Food for Travel

Some of the time, it's simpler to simply maintain a strategic distance from the problems of cooking by and large.

One case of this is if your hiking or voyaging. Non-perishable foods permit you to abstain from building a fire or pulling a compact oven.

This can assist spare with weighting or space.

Besides, for exploring, you are ordinarily depleted before the day's over. You simply need to set up camp, eat, unwind, and head to sleep.

So why not make the devouring procedure as basic and easy as could reasonably be expected. It's a task to prepare a feast when your vitality is drained, and your stomach is thundering.

- For Donation

Most food drives, banks approach explicitly for "non perishable food things". They need foods they can reserve, transport, and serve without agonizing over refrigeration.

Would you be able to envision attempting to take care of thousands of destitute and starving individuals new servings of mixed greens? It would probably ruin before they could serve it.

One of the staples of food gift is canned foods – they are quite often a savvy blessing. However, I urge you not to simply give canned food that you've never eaten in light of the fact that it's gross. Give taste and sound canned foods.

CHAPTER TWO

BELOW ARE LISTS OF NON PERISHABLE FOODS

- Beef Jerky

- Granola Bars

- Dried Pasta (ramen noodles, macaroni, spaghetti, and so on.)

- Trail Mix (particularly the nuts)

- Dry Rice and Beans (Canned Foods (meats, vegetables, natural products, soups)

- Freeze Dried Meals Oatmeal

- Peanut Butter

- Apple Sauce

- Coffee Beans

- Pancake Mix

- Sugar

- Syrup

- Vegetable Oil

- Crackers (hardtack)

- MRE's

- Pemmican)

- Powdered Milk

- Dried Fruits

- Most Dry Spices

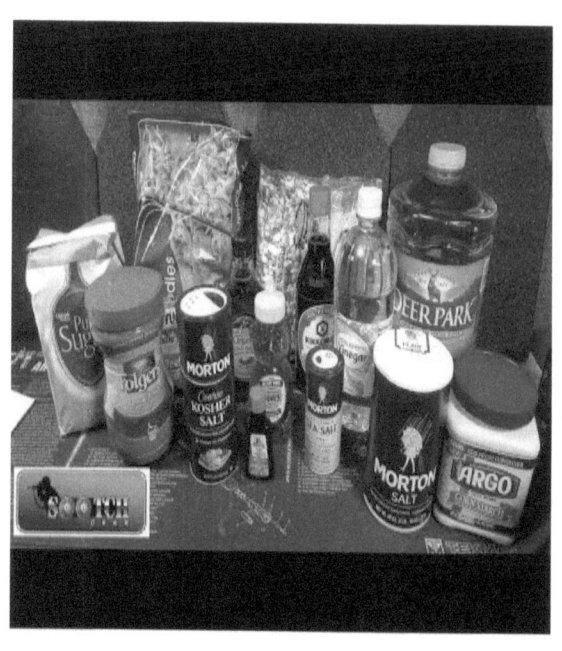

WHERE TO BUY NON-PERISHABLE FOODS

You can get numerous non-perishable things from your nearby supermarket.

Nutty spread, wafers, nectar, and so on are for the most part promptly accessible to pull off the rack. Be that as it may, one sort of food that progressively hard to track down at the merchant is Freeze Dried Foods.

These non-perishable foods are made by strength producers. Be that as it may, you won't locate a wide determination of freeze dried foods in your nearby supermarket.

They sell them for the most part at outdoor supplies stores or on the web.

So why make a special effort to put resources into freeze-dried foods? Since they are the best food for preparedness and readiness.

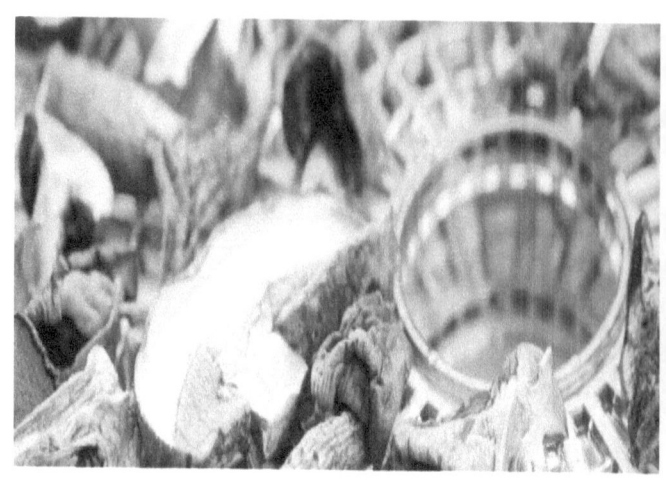

FOODS WHICH DON'T REQUIRE REFRIGERATION OR COOKING

At the point when the force is down, your cooler and electric oven won't work. In the event that you are preparing for power blackouts or other catastrophe, at that point I suggest getting a little oven. I for one like propane hiking ovens best, yet there are a lot of different choices as well.

• Oatmeal with freeze-dried organic products: Soak 5-10 minutes or until wanted non-abrasiveness. Dried out organic products take any longer to mellow.

• Instant pureed potatoes

• Ramen: Soak 15-30 minutes or until it is totally delicate. Pastas tragically should be cooked to separate the proteins.

• Couscous: Soak 20-30 minutes

• Instant rice: Soak around 2 hours.

• Hummus blend: Soak 10 minutes.

- Cream soups (no noodles or bits of vegetables): Soak 10-30 minutes.

- Rice noodles: Soak 60 minutes.

- Freeze dried hiking dinners (no noodles or pasta): Most hiking suppers are intended to be cooked, so can't be made along these lines. In any case, the ones with no kind of pasta in them can for the most part be cold splashed.

CHAPTER THREE

HOW TO MAKE PERISHABLE FOODS INTO NON-PERISHABLE FOODS

Making a food non-perishable comes down to diminishing microorganisms' capacity to develop.

Microscopic organisms are a natural substance; it's alive. So simply like you and me, it has essential endurance needs.

Microbes/Bacteria needs the following to endure:

- Mild Temperature Ranges

- Air (oxygen)

- Moisture (water)

- Food

Presently – before we begin blocking microorganisms – we can't obstruct the keep going thing on the rundown – Food. Why? Since food is the thing that we are attempting to ensure. Take out the food source invalidates the point!

However, on the off chance that you hinder any of the other key fixings, you can decrease microbes' malicious designs to ruin your food.

Temperature Control

The vast majority of us as of now forestall food decay each day utilizing coolers and coolers. Cold temperatures lessen microbes' capacity to endure or flourish.

In freezing cold temps, it bites the dust. In cooler temps, it can endure however is more fragile and doesn't flourish.

Note: Before power and refrigeration came – there were root basements and coolers. Not close to as helpful however the standards were the equivalent. Lower temperatures protect food longer.

Suffocation

Another approach to battle food ruining microbes is to evacuate oxygen.

Microbes needs oxygen to endure. So by utilizing vacuum fixing, or oxygen safeguards, or potentially mylar packs, you can store food separate from oxygen.

Evacuate the Moisture

At long last, microscopic organisms needs water (for example dampness) to endure. In the event that you expel most or all the dampness in food, microbes won't ruin it.

In any case, as we'll see in the blink of an eye, there is a major contrast between dried out foods (diminished dampness) and freeze-dried food (close to zero dampness).

So now we should go over a couple of the more regular ways individuals lessen microscopic organisms capacity to ruin their foods.

Canning

Once tried approach to protect food is canning, particularly your additional nursery produce.

Basically, canning is placing veggies into sealable jars with fluid. At that point utilizing a warming and cooling procedure to make a vacuum (for example no air).

Why? Since simply like us, microscopic organisms need air to endure. So with no oxygen, microorganisms can't get by to annihilate your canned foods.

Freeze Drying

Freeze drying foods is a procedure that expels almost all the dampness out of food. In any case, does as such in a way that doesn't harm the food.

Keep in mind, dampness is a key element for bacterial development. So by expelling all dampness, you're disposing of bacterial development on the food.

Freeze drying leaves the food in a state ready to acknowledge and reconstitute dampness. As a rule, you simply need to add fluids to the food and permit it to reabsorb dampness. With certain suppers, you add bubbling water to reconstitute and prepare the food.

Be that as it may, freeze drying all alone is either mind boggling or costly.

On the off chance that you attempt to make your own freeze dryer – it will be a confused building venture. Indeed, it very well may be done however at the expense of a great deal of time and vitality.

The other method to make your own freeze dried food is to purchase a home freeze dryer.

Drying out

Drying out food is to some degree like freeze drying yet it's not close to as viable. Both decrease dampness yet in immeasurably various manners. Rather than utilizing vacuum chambers and dried ice, you simply use warmth and air development to evacuate dampness.

The mix of warmth and air dries out the foods.

Also, once more, absence of dampness is one demonstrated system to end or decrease the ruining procedure.

On a par with this sounds – getting dried out isn't close to as successful as freeze drying. Sure you can transform a perishable apple into non-perishable apple chips. It's certainly better than nothing and will forestall bacterial development. Yet, dried out foods won't a decades ago like freeze drying.

Freeze Drying VS Dehydrating

One approach to consider drying out versus freeze-drying is to contrast it with a Refrigerator versus a Freezer.

A fridge eases back bacterial development however doesn't totally dispense with it. A cooler disposes of bacterial development. So getting dried out is somewhat similar to refrigeration (eases back the development) while freeze drying is increasingly similar to a cooler (wipes out all development).

In any case, hold up drying is better than coolers since it needn't bother with a steady progression of power!

Back to drying out – the uplifting news is, drying out is both simple to do yourself and incredibly reasonable. You can most likely beginning getting dried out products of the soil today utilizing devices you effectively own.

All you need is one of the following:

1.   A customary broiler (low warmth – air out the entryway)

2.   A food dehydrator, or

3.   A DIY terrace dehydrator (utilizing wind and sun)

CHAPTER FOUR

HEALTHY NON PERISHABLE FOOD

Some non-perishable foods are more beneficial than others.

For instance, MRE (suppers prepared to eat) are NOT known for their wellbeing.

They're pressed with calories to give warriors in the field a lot of vitality. Be that as it may, in case you're eating MRE's and not practicing a lot, don't' be astounded on the off chance that you begin pressing on the pounds.

Soups additionally will in general have a great deal of sodium – so make an effort not to eat canned soup for each feast!

In any case, nuts (like Almonds) are exceptionally sound for you. Beans are a sound type of protein.

And keeping in mind that canned vegetables don't taste as new as nursery veggies, they're as yet a solid non perishable food thing.

Along these lines, keep your store sound by settling on insightful non perishable food decisions.

NON-PERISHABLE FOOD FOR HURRICANES

Individuals will in general get some information about non perishable food-identified with typhoons.

Why hurricanes and not different crises?

I believe this is on the grounds that storms or hurricanes are a calamity you typically observe seeking days early. So when a tropical storm begins turning into a reality, individuals begin inquiring about their food choices.

Different crises happen quick and unexpectantly – like tornados, quakes, out of control fires, and so forth. You don't a similar measure of timely notification for these fiascos…

All things considered, your non-perishable food for storms is the same than some other sort of crisis. Calories will be calories when the markets are down and out.

In any case, perhaps you should include a couple of additional jars of spinach (like Popeye) in the event that you need the additional solidarity to face the hardship. Something else and the foods in the non-perishable foods models recorded above will accomplish for your typhoon prep list.

Simply ensure you keep the non-perishable foods in a safe secure area. In the event that your home is decimated by the tropical storm and your food was in your upstairs wash room

So attempt to store the non-perishable foods (for example prepper food) in a cellar or as secure an area as could reasonably be expected.

CHAPTER FIVE

FOODS THAT CAN BE FROZEN

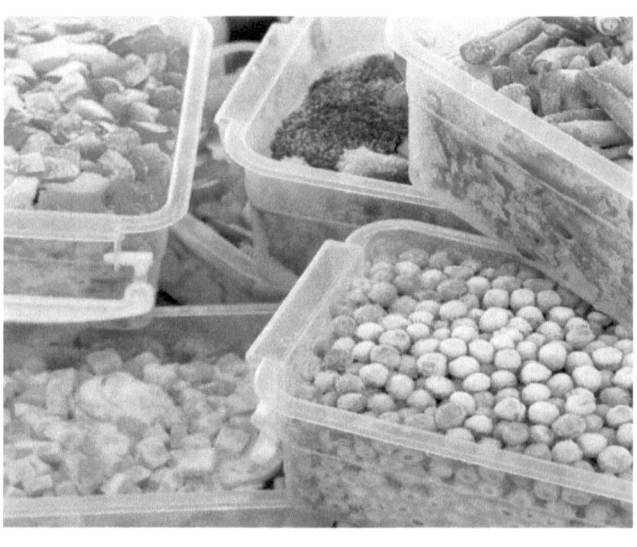

Another answer for defeat the terminated date of a portion of the item is to freeze them. Obviously not all the items can be solidified. We offer you now an impressive rundown of various items that can be utilized in a period on account of the cooler. They will remain new for quite a while.

Freeze dried foods are famous among explorers in view of their light weight and movability.

Freeze dried foods and prepared to-eat freeze dried suppers are made for long haul stockpiling — with certain items flaunting a 30-year taste ensure.

Numerous organizations freeze-dried suppers that are sound as well as suit explicit dietary examples.

Step by step instructions on how to freeze fruits and vegetables

- Bread
- Stocks, Pestos and Tomato Sauces
- Butter

- Cheese
- Doughs and Batters
- Eggs (broke into ice 3D square plate)
- Fruits and Vegetables
- Herbs (freeze in little ice 3D square plate with olive oil)
- Meats (cooked and crude including bacon and lunch meat)
- Tortillas

Drink Non-Perishable Foods

Plant-based beverages like soy milk bundled in adaptable materials, including plastic, paper, and aluminum, comparably last as long as 10 months, while canned coconut milk keeps as long as 5 years at room temperature.

Rack stable and plant-based milks can be utilized when refrigeration isn't accessible. Powdered milk is a decent other option, with an expected time span of usability of 3–5 years when kept in a cool, dull spot. It very well may be reconstituted with clean water in little segments varying.

Tea and coffee is one of the non perishable beverages

- Coffee
- dissipated milk
- flavorings for water
- Gatorade
- juice
- apple
- cranberry
- fruit juice
- grape
- vegetable juice
- lemonade

- dinner substitution drinks like Ensure
- nondairy milk, for example, canned coconut milk
- powdered beverage blends
- powdered hot cocoa
- powdered milk
- rack stable milk
- tea sacks
- water
- Classes

THE END